THE SKIN SYMPHONY

BREAKING FREE FROM ECZEMA

Dr. Rachel Thompson

Copyright

TABLE OF CONTENT

INTRODUCTION

Eczema, a term encompassing various inflammatory skin conditions, has become increasingly prevalent across diverse demographics. In this introductory chapter, we embark on a journey to demystify eczema, offering readers a nuanced understanding of its multifaceted nature.

At its core, eczema is more than a dermatological ailment—it represents a complex interplay of genetic, environmental, and immunological factors. We delve into the different types of eczema, including the well-known atopic dermatitis, contact dermatitis, and the less common but equally impactful varieties such as dyshidrotic eczema. By elucidating the causes and triggers, readers gain insight into the intricate web of elements that contribute to the onset and exacerbation of eczematous conditions.

Moving beyond a clinical lens, we explore the nuanced manifestations of eczema, unraveling the diverse symptoms that individuals may experience. This chapter serves as a diagnostic guide, equipping readers with the knowledge to identify eczema across various age groups. The importance of seeking medical evaluation and undergoing diagnostic tests is underscored, laying the foundation for subsequent sections on effective management and treatment.

As we embark on this exploration, the introduction sets the stage for an empowering journey. Readers are encouraged to navigate the complexities of eczema armed with knowledge, fostering a sense of agency in managing their condition. The forthcoming chapters promise a holistic approach, encompassing medical interventions, lifestyle adjustments, and the emotional terrain that individuals with eczema navigate. In essence, this introduction not only defines the scope of the book but also invites readers into a space where understanding meets empowerment in the realm of eczema management.

Brief Overview of its Prevalence

Eczema's prevalence has evolved into a significant global health concern, impacting millions of individuals across diverse age groups and demographics. As we embark on a comprehensive exploration of eczema in this book, understanding its prevalence is paramount to grasp the magnitude of its influence on public health.

Atopic dermatitis, one of the most common forms of eczema, has witnessed a steady rise in prevalence over the past few decades. This chronic inflammatory skin condition extends its reach to both children and adults, with early onset often observed in childhood. Statistics reveal a substantial increase in reported cases, emphasizing the need for heightened awareness and effective management strategies.

Beyond atopic dermatitis, eczema encompasses a spectrum of conditions, each presenting its unique challenges. Contact dermatitis, triggered by exposure to specific substances, affects individuals in occupational and non-occupational settings. Dyshidrotic eczema, characterized by blistering on the hands and feet, adds another layer of complexity to the prevalence landscape.

Environmental factors play a pivotal role in the prevalence of eczema. Changing climates, increased pollution, and exposure to allergens contribute to the escalation of eczematous conditions worldwide. Geographical variations in prevalence underscore the intricate interplay between genetic predisposition and environmental triggers.

This brief overview illuminates eczema's ubiquity, emphasizing its relevance not only in individual lives but also in the broader context of public health. By recognizing the widespread impact of eczema, we set the stage for a deeper exploration into its causes, manifestations, and effective management strategies. As we navigate the pages ahead, this awareness forms a cornerstone, guiding readers through a comprehensive understanding of eczema's prevalence and the imperative for informed, compassionate approaches to address this prevalent dermatological challenge.

CHAPTER 1

UNDERSTANDING ECZEMA

Understanding eczema involves unraveling the intricate tapestry of factors that contribute to this complex and often chronic skin condition. At its essence, eczema is not a singular ailment but a collective term for a group of inflammatory skin disorders characterized by redness, itching, and various skin lesions. To comprehend eczema is to navigate its diverse types, explore its origins, and appreciate the multifaceted nature of its manifestation. First and foremost, eczema manifests in different forms, each presenting unique challenges. Atopic dermatitis, the most prevalent type, is often linked to genetic predispositions and immune system dysregulation. Contact dermatitis, on the other hand, emerges as a result of direct contact with irritants or allergens, making it more predictable in its triggers. Dyshidrotic eczema, distinguished by blisters on the hands and feet, adds another layer of complexity to the spectrum.

The causes of eczema are manifold, intertwining genetic, environmental, and immunological elements. Understanding the genetic predisposition to atopic dermatitis sheds light on the hereditary nature of some eczematous conditions. Environmental factors, such as exposure to allergens, irritants, and climatic changes, contribute significantly to the onset and exacerbation of eczema.

As we delve into understanding eczema, it becomes evident that its manifestations extend beyond the skin. The intricate interplay between genetic susceptibility, environmental triggers, and immune responses requires a holistic approach to decipher. This chapter lays the groundwork for comprehending the complexities of eczema, preparing readers for the subsequent exploration of diagnostic approaches, management strategies, and the impact of eczema on various aspects of life. In essence, understanding eczema is not merely unraveling a dermatological mystery but embarking on a journey to grasp the intricacies of an ailment that reverberates across the realms of genetics, environment, and individual well-being.

Types of Eczema

Eczema encompasses a spectrum of skin disorders, each presenting unique characteristics and challenges. Understanding the various types of eczema is essential for accurate diagnosis and tailored management. This chapter delves into the diverse manifestations of eczema, shedding light on the distinct features that define each type.

- **Atopic Dermatitis:** Atopic dermatitis stands out as the most prevalent and well-known form of eczema. It often begins in infancy and is characterized by red, itchy rashes. Genetic factors play a significant role, with a family history of atopic conditions like asthma and allergic rhinitis often observed.
- **Contact Dermatitis:** Contact dermatitis results from direct contact with irritants or allergens. Occupational exposure, skincare products, and certain metals can trigger this type of eczema. It manifests as redness, itching, and sometimes blistering in the affected area.
- **Dyshidrotic Eczema:** Dyshidrotic eczema primarily affects the palms of the hands and soles of the feet. It is characterized by small, itchy blisters and can be

triggered by factors like stress, allergies, or exposure to certain metals.

- **Nummular Eczema:** Nummular eczema, also known as discoid eczema, presents as coin-shaped patches of irritated skin. These circular lesions can be intensely itchy and may result from dry skin, injury, or allergic reactions.

- **Seborrheic Dermatitis:** Seborrheic dermatitis commonly affects areas with high oil production, such as the scalp, face, and chest. It results in red, scaly, and sometimes greasy skin. While the exact cause is unclear, factors like yeast overgrowth and genetics may contribute.

Causes and Triggers

Edema, characterized by the abnormal accumulation of fluid in body tissues, is a complex condition influenced by a myriad of causes and triggers. Distinguishing between these factors is crucial for a comprehensive understanding, accurate diagnosis, and effective treatment. Causes are often underlying conditions or systemic issues that lead to the development of edema, while triggers are external factors or events that exacerbate or provoke existing edema. Let's explore each category in detail.

Causes of Edema:

1. **Imbalance in Fluid Regulation:** The circulatory system orchestrates fluid movement, maintaining equilibrium through capillary filtration. Elevated hydrostatic pressure within blood vessels, as seen in congestive heart failure, can result in fluid backup and subsequent leakage into tissues, leading to edema. Conversely, a decrease in osmotic pressure due to conditions like liver disease or malnutrition contributes to edema by reducing the proteins, especially albumin, needed to maintain osmotic balance.

2. **Lymphatic System Dysfunction:** The lymphatic system, responsible for draining excess fluid and supporting immune function, can be compromised. Lymphedema, often arising from surgical removal of lymph nodes or other lymphatic disorders, manifests as localized fluid accumulation, leading to swelling. The inability of the lymphatic system to efficiently drain fluids exacerbates fluid retention, contributing significantly to the development of edema.

3. **Inflammation**: Inflammatory processes trigger increased permeability of blood vessels, allowing fluids and immune cells to move into inflamed tissues. While inflammation is a part of the body's defense mechanism, prolonged or excessive inflammation can result in persistent edema. Conditions like rheumatoid arthritis or infections induce edema as a secondary effect. Inflammatory mediators, including histamines, can dilate blood vessels, contributing to increased permeability and fluid accumulation in tissues.

4. **Hormonal Changes:** Hormonal fluctuations, particularly during the menstrual cycle or pregnancy, play a role in fluid homeostasis. Imbalances in hormones can lead to water retention, contributing to edema. Premenstrual syndrome (PMS) often involves fluid retention as a symptom. Medications that influence hormonal levels, such as oral contraceptives or corticosteroids, can also result in edema as a side effect. Estrogen, in particular, has been implicated in promoting sodium and water retention, affecting overall fluid balance.

5. **Kidney Dysfunction:** Renal dysfunction significantly contributes to systemic edema. The kidneys, crucial

for regulating fluid balance, filter waste and excess fluids from the blood. Conditions like chronic kidney disease or acute kidney injury compromise this filtration process, leading to inadequate fluid excretion and generalized edema. Sodium retention, often associated with impaired kidney function, contributes to increased fluid retention throughout the body.

6. **Local Obstruction to Fluid Drainage:** Tumors or masses, benign or malignant, can obstruct the normal flow of fluids by compressing lymphatic vessels or blood vessels. This local obstruction hinders efficient drainage, resulting in swelling in the affected area. Surgical interventions or radiation therapy aimed at addressing tumors may contribute to lymphatic system disruption, complicating the development of edema.

7. **Inactivity and Lifestyle Factors:** Prolonged inactivity, such as standing or sitting for extended periods, contributes to venous stasis and edema. Gravity impedes the efficient return of blood and lymphatic fluid to the heart, resulting in swelling, particularly in the lower extremities. Certain occupations that require prolonged standing may predispose individuals to this

type of edema. Lifestyle factors such as a sedentary lifestyle or obesity can contribute to fluid retention and edema, as lack of physical activity diminishes the natural pumping action of muscles aiding venous return.

Triggers of Edema:

1. **Infection and Acute Inflammatory Events:** Acute inflammatory events, such as infections or injuries, can trigger edema. In response to inflammation, blood vessels become more permeable, allowing fluids and immune cells to move into the affected area. This localized edema is a protective response but can become problematic if inflammation persists.

2. **Temperature and Climate:** Extreme temperatures, especially heat, can contribute to fluid retention and exacerbate edema. In warmer climates, individuals may experience increased swelling, as heat can dilate blood vessels and impact fluid balance.

3. **Dietary Factors:** High-sodium diets can lead to water retention and exacerbate edema. Excessive salt intake can contribute to fluid imbalance, as the body retains water to dilute the increased sodium concentration.

4. **Medication Side Effects:** Certain medications, including antihypertensives, nonsteroidal anti-inflammatory drugs (NSAIDs), and corticosteroids, can cause fluid retention and edema as side effects. Understanding the potential impact of medications is crucial in managing edema.

5. **Allergies**: Allergic reactions can induce edema, particularly in the form of angioedema. This condition involves swelling in the deeper layers of the skin, often around the eyes and lips, and can be triggered by allergens like certain foods or insect stings.

6. **Trauma and Injury:** Physical trauma or injury, such as fractures or sprains, can result in localized edema. The body's response to injury includes increased blood flow and vessel permeability, leading to swelling in the affected area.

7. **Hormonal Fluctuations in Women:** Hormonal fluctuations during the menstrual cycle can act as triggers for edema in some women. The hormonal changes that occur during different phases of the menstrual cycle can influence fluid retention.

8. **Surgical Interventions:** Surgeries, especially those involving lymph node removal or vascular procedures, can disrupt the normal flow of fluids and trigger localized or systemic edema. Post-surgical edema is a common occurrence and requires careful management.

Understanding the intricate interplay between these causes and triggers is essential for healthcare professionals to formulate a precise diagnosis and tailored treatment plan. The dynamic nature of edema necessitates a comprehensive approach that addresses both the underlying conditions leading to edema and the external factors that can exacerbate or trigger its manifestation. Advances in medical research will likely continue to refine our understanding of edema, paving the way for more targeted and effective therapeutic interventions.

CHAPTER TWO

CLINICAL PRESENTATION

The clinical presentation of eczema encompasses a diverse array of symptoms and physical manifestations that vary depending on the specific type of eczema and individual factors. Understanding these clinical aspects is pivotal for accurate diagnosis and effective management of this complex skin condition.

1. **Rash and Inflammation:** A hallmark of eczema is the development of a red, inflamed rash on the skin. This rash can appear in different patterns, ranging from small, raised bumps to larger, irregular patches. The inflammatory response is a key feature, often accompanied by itching, which can be intense and persistent.

2. **Itching (Pruritus):** Itching is a defining characteristic of eczema and is often the most distressing symptom for individuals. The urge to scratch can be overwhelming, leading to skin damage, increased inflammation, and a potential vicious cycle of itching and scratching.

3. **Dry and Flaky Skin:** Eczematous skin tends to be dry and may exhibit flakiness or scaling. The compromised skin barrier in eczema reduces the ability to retain moisture, contributing to dryness. Maintaining proper skin hydration is a key aspect of managing eczema.

4. **Blisters (Dyshidrotic Eczema):** In the case of dyshidrotic eczema, small, fluid-filled blisters may develop on the hands and feet. These blisters can be intensely itchy and contribute to the unique clinical presentation of this particular type of eczema.

5. **Cracking and Oozing:** Severe eczema may lead to skin fissures or cracks, which can ooze fluid. This occurs as a result of the compromised skin barrier, allowing irritants to penetrate and exacerbate inflammation. Oozing lesions can increase the risk of secondary infections.

6. **Lichenification**: Chronic scratching and rubbing can result in lichenification, a condition where the skin becomes thickened and hardened. This response is the skin's attempt to protect itself from ongoing irritation but can contribute to further complications.

7. **Variable Presentation of Nummular Eczema:** Nummular eczema, characterized by coin-shaped patches, presents with distinct circular lesions. These patches can be intensely itchy and may have a crusted or scaly appearance.

8. **Seborrheic Dermatitis Features:** Seborrheic dermatitis often affects areas rich in sebaceous glands, such as the scalp, face, and chest. It manifests with red, scaly patches and may involve the eyebrows and hairline.

Understanding the clinical presentation of eczema extends beyond recognizing visible symptoms; it involves appreciating the impact on the individual's quality of life. The constant itching, discomfort, and potential complications demand a holistic approach to management, addressing both the physical and psychological aspects of this dermatological condition. Healthcare providers play a crucial role in evaluating these clinical features, tailoring treatment plans, and offering support to enhance the well-being of individuals living with eczema.

Eczema in Different Age Groups

Identifying eczema in different age groups involves recognizing variations in clinical presentation, triggers, and the impact on quality of life. Eczema can manifest differently as individuals progress through infancy, childhood, adolescence, and adulthood, necessitating a nuanced understanding for accurate diagnosis and effective management.

- **Infants**: Eczema often makes its debut in infancy, typically appearing on the face, scalp, and extensor surfaces of the extremities. The rash may be red, scaly, and accompanied by intense itching. In infants, the constant rubbing and scratching can result in crusted lesions. Diaper area involvement is common, and careful assessment is crucial to differentiate eczema from other pediatric dermatological conditions.

- **Children**: As children grow, eczema commonly affects flexural folds such as the elbows and knees. Itchy, red patches may develop, and the condition can significantly impact a child's daily activities and sleep. Allergies, environmental factors, and genetic predispositions play key roles in pediatric eczema, requiring a comprehensive evaluation for optimal management.

- **Adolescents**: During adolescence, hormonal changes may influence the presentation of eczema. Stressors related to puberty, academic pressures, and social dynamics can exacerbate symptoms. Adolescents with eczema may also face unique challenges in self-esteem and body image, underscoring the importance of addressing the emotional impact of the condition.

- **Adults**: In adulthood, eczema can persist or recur, with variations in affected areas. Flexural folds, hands, and face remain common sites, but eczema may also appear on the neck, wrists, and ankles. Adult-onset eczema may be associated with workplace exposures, stress, and changes in climate or lifestyle.

- **Older Adults:** Eczema in older adults may exhibit distinctive features due to age-related changes in the skin. Reduced skin elasticity, dryness, and comorbidities may influence the clinical presentation. Management considerations include adapting to the unique skin needs of older individuals and addressing potential interactions with other medical conditions. Identifying eczema in different age groups requires a holistic approach, considering both physical and psychosocial factors. Healthcare professionals play a crucial role in evaluating symptoms, conducting thorough assessments, and tailoring management plans to meet the specific needs of individuals at different life stages. By recognizing the age-specific nuances of eczema, practitioners can enhance diagnostic accuracy and provide comprehensive care to improve the overall well-being of patients across the lifespan.

CHAPTER THREE

DIAGNOSING ECZEMA

Diagnosing eczema involves a combination of clinical evaluation, patient history, and, in some cases, additional tests. Given the diverse types and presentations of eczema, a comprehensive approach is essential to accurately identify the specific condition and tailor an effective treatment plan.

> **Medical Evaluation:** The diagnostic process often begins with a thorough medical evaluation by a healthcare professional, such as a dermatologist. Medical evaluation plays a pivotal role in the diagnosis of eczema, providing healthcare professionals with crucial insights into the nature and extent of the condition. A comprehensive assessment involves a combination of clinical observation, patient

history, and sometimes additional tests to ensure an accurate diagnosis.

➢ **Clinical Observation:** The cornerstone of the medical evaluation is the physical examination of the affected skin. Healthcare professionals, often dermatologists, meticulously examine the skin for characteristic signs of eczema. These may include redness, inflammation, dryness, and a variety of rash patterns. The distribution of the rash, such as its presence in flexural folds or other specific areas, can offer valuable diagnostic clues.

➢ **Symptom Assessment:** A thorough evaluation of eczema symptoms involves assessing the appearance, distribution, and characteristics of skin lesions. Common symptoms include redness, dryness, intense itching, and the development of papules, vesicles, or oozing lesions. The distribution of these symptoms on the body can vary, with certain areas like the flexor surfaces of joints being commonly affected. The severity of symptoms is a crucial aspect of the evaluation. Healthcare professionals often use standardized tools, such as the Eczema Area and Severity Index (EASI) or the SCORing Atopic Dermatitis (SCORAD) index, to quantify the extent and intensity of eczema lesions. This objective measurement aids in monitoring changes over time and assessing treatment efficacy.

- ➢ **Patient History:** A detailed medical history is crucial in evaluating eczema. Healthcare providers inquire about the onset of symptoms, family history of skin conditions or allergies, and any known triggers or exacerbating factors. Understanding the patient's overall health, previous treatments, and lifestyle factors provides valuable insights into the nature and potential causes of eczema.Information about the patient's occupation, exposure to irritants or allergens, dietary habits, and stress levels can be particularly relevant. Additionally, inquiring about other allergic conditions, such as hay fever or asthma, is essential since eczema often coexists with these allergic tendencies, a phenomenon known as the atopic triad.

- ➢ **Differential Diagnosis:** Given the diversity of dermatological conditions, differentiating eczema from other skin disorders is essential. The healthcare professional considers potential mimicking conditions, such as psoriasis or contact dermatitis, to arrive at a precise diagnosis. In some cases, additional tests, like a skin biopsy, may be recommended to confirm the diagnosis or rule out other skin disorders.

> **Collaboration and Specialized Input:** Collaboration with other specialists may be warranted in certain situations. For instance, if allergies are suspected to be triggering eczema, consultation with an allergist can provide valuable insights. This interdisciplinary approach ensures a holistic understanding of the patient's condition and contributes to more effective diagnosis and management.

In conclusion, the medical evaluation for eczema is a comprehensive process that combines clinical observation, patient history, and, when necessary, additional tests. This thorough assessment lays the foundation for a precise diagnosis, enabling healthcare providers to tailor treatment plans to the specific needs of each individual and improve overall outcomes in managing eczema.

Diagnostic Tests and Procedures

Diagnostic tests and procedures play a crucial role in the comprehensive evaluation of eczema, helping healthcare professionals confirm the diagnosis, rule out other skin conditions, and gain insights into potential triggers. While the clinical presentation is often indicative, certain situations may warrant additional tests to refine the diagnostic process.

1. **Patch Testing:** Patch testing is a valuable tool, especially in cases where contact dermatitis is suspected as a trigger for eczema. This procedure involves applying small amounts of common allergens to the skin using adhesive patches. The patches remain in place for a set period, usually 48 hours, after which the skin is examined for any allergic reactions. Patch testing helps identify specific substances, such as metals, fragrances, or preservatives, that may be contributing to eczema flares.

2. **Skin Biopsy:** In cases where the clinical presentation is ambiguous or when healthcare professionals need to differentiate between eczema and other skin disorders, a skin biopsy may be recommended. During this procedure, a small sample of affected skin is removed and examined under a microscope. Skin biopsy findings can provide valuable insights into the histological characteristics of the skin, helping to confirm the diagnosis or identify other dermatological conditions.

3. **Blood Tests:** While blood tests are not routinely used for diagnosing eczema itself, they can be instrumental in specific situations. Blood tests may be conducted to assess immune system function, particularly in cases where the healthcare professional suspects underlying immunological issues. Identifying immune system abnormalities can guide treatment decisions and shed light on the potential systemic aspects of eczematous conditions.

4. **Allergy Testing:** Allergy testing may be considered, especially in cases where specific allergens are suspected triggers for eczema. Various allergy testing methods, including skin prick tests or blood tests, can help identify sensitivities to common allergens such as pollen, dust mites, animal dander, and certain foods. Managing and avoiding identified allergens can contribute to reducing eczema flares in individuals with allergic triggers.

5. **Skin Cultures:** In cases where secondary bacterial or fungal infections are suspected due to oozing or crusted lesions, a healthcare professional may perform skin cultures. This involves collecting a sample from the affected area for laboratory analysis to identify the

specific pathogens causing the infection. Treatment plans can then be adjusted to target the underlying infection alongside eczema management.

6. **Phototesting**: For certain types of eczema, such as photocontact dermatitis, phototesting may be employed. This involves exposing the skin to specific wavelengths of ultraviolet (UV) light to identify if light exposure contributes to eczema flares. Phototesting can help tailor recommendations for sun protection and guide management strategies.

7. **Environmental and Patch Elimination Tests:** In situations where environmental factors are suspected triggers, healthcare professionals may recommend environmental or patch elimination tests. These involve temporarily avoiding or removing potential triggers, such as specific skincare products or fabrics, to observe whether symptoms improve. Reintroduction of these elements can help confirm their role in eczema flares.

8. **History of Atopic Conditions:** While not a formal diagnostic test, a comprehensive history-taking is a critical aspect of the diagnostic process. Inquiring about a patient's personal and family history of atopic

conditions, such as asthma, hay fever, or other allergies, provides important context. The presence of these conditions can contribute to the likelihood of developing eczema.

In conclusion, diagnostic tests and procedures in eczema evaluation serve as valuable tools to enhance accuracy and tailor treatment approaches. The selection of specific tests depends on the individual's clinical presentation, suspected triggers, and the need for further clarification. By combining clinical observation with appropriate diagnostic measures, healthcare professionals can develop personalized management plans that address the unique aspects of each individual's eczematous condition.

CHAPTER FOUR

MANAGEMENT STRATEGIES

Effective management strategies for eczema focus on alleviating symptoms, reducing inflammation, and preventing flare-ups. A holistic approach that combines skincare practices, lifestyle modifications, and, when necessary, medical interventions can significantly improve the quality of life for individuals with eczema.

1. **Skincare Routine:** A consistent and gentle skincare routine is fundamental in managing eczema. Use mild, fragrance-free cleansers and moisturizers to hydrate the skin regularly. Avoid hot water and opt for lukewarm baths or showers. Pat the skin dry instead of rubbing to minimize irritation.

2. **Moisturization**: Regular moisturization is a cornerstone of eczema management. Applying an

emollient or hypoallergenic moisturizer helps maintain the skin barrier, reducing dryness and itchiness. Moisturizers should be applied immediately after bathing to lock in moisture.

3. **Avoiding Triggers:** Identifying and avoiding triggers is crucial for preventing eczema flare-ups. This may involve patch testing to identify specific allergens, as well as recognizing environmental factors like certain fabrics, skincare products, or exposure to irritants that contribute to skin irritation.

Tropical treatments

Topical treatments are a cornerstone in the management of eczema, providing targeted relief by addressing inflammation, itching, and skin barrier function. These medications are applied directly to the affected skin, offering a localized approach to control symptoms. Understanding the types of topical treatments available and their proper usage is crucial for effective eczema management.

1. **Topical Corticosteroids:** Topical corticosteroids are commonly prescribed to reduce inflammation and

itching during eczema flare-ups. They work by suppressing the immune response and alleviating symptoms. Corticosteroids come in varying strengths, with milder formulations suitable for sensitive areas like the face and stronger ones for thicker skin on the body. It's important to use them as directed by a healthcare professional to minimize side effects, such as thinning of the skin.

2. **Topical Calcineurin Inhibitors:** Calcineurin inhibitors, such as tacrolimus and pimecrolimus, are another class of topical medications used to control inflammation in eczema. These agents are particularly useful for sensitive areas like the face and are often recommended when corticosteroids may not be suitable for long-term use.

3. **Topical Phosphodiesterase-4 (PDE4) Inhibitors:** Crisaborole, a topical PDE4 inhibitor, is a newer addition to eczema treatment. It helps reduce inflammation and is often prescribed for mild to moderate eczema. Unlike corticosteroids, PDE4 inhibitors are non-steroidal, offering an alternative for those concerned about potential corticosteroid side effects.

4. **Emollients and Moisturizers:** While not traditional medications, emollients and moisturizers are essential components of eczema management. These products help hydrate the skin, maintain the skin barrier, and reduce dryness. Regular use of fragrance-free moisturizers, especially after bathing, is crucial for individuals with eczema to prevent flare-ups.

5. **Topical Antibiotics:** In cases where eczema lesions are secondarily infected due to scratching and compromised skin integrity, topical antibiotics may be prescribed. These medications target bacterial overgrowth, aiding in the healing process.

6. **Wet Wrap Therapy:** Wet wrap therapy involves applying a damp layer over emollients or prescription creams, followed by a dry layer. This technique enhances the absorption of moisturizers and medications, providing additional relief during acute episodes.

7. **Topical Antihistamines:** Topical antihistamines are less commonly used than oral forms but may be recommended in certain situations. They can help alleviate itching by blocking histamine receptors in the skin.

8. **Compliance and Follow-up:** Effective use of topical treatments requires adherence to prescribed regimens and regular follow-ups with healthcare professionals. Monitoring the skin's response, adjusting treatment plans as needed, and addressing any concerns or side effects contribute to successful eczema management.

Individual responses to topical treatments can vary, and healthcare professionals work closely with patients to determine the most suitable approach. A tailored regimen, considering the severity and location of eczema, helps individuals achieve better control of symptoms while minimizing potential side effects associated with prolonged medication use.

Systemic medications

Systemic medications play a crucial role in the management of eczema, particularly in cases where topical treatments may be insufficient to control widespread or severe symptoms. These medications are administered internally, affecting the entire body to address the underlying causes of inflammation and immune dysregulation associated with eczema.

1. **Oral Corticosteroids:** Oral corticosteroids are potent anti-inflammatory medications that may be prescribed for short-term use during severe eczema flare-ups. They work by suppressing the immune response and reducing inflammation throughout the body. However, due to potential side effects such as weight gain, increased blood pressure, and bone density loss, long-term use is generally avoided.

2. **Oral Immunosuppressants:** Immunosuppressive medications, such as cyclosporine or methotrexate, are prescribed for individuals with moderate to severe eczema that hasn't responded well to other treatments. These medications work by suppressing the immune system, helping to reduce inflammation and control symptoms. Regular monitoring and follow-ups are essential to manage potential side effects, including effects on kidney function and liver toxicity.

3. **Oral JAK Inhibitors:** Janus kinase (JAK) inhibitors are a newer class of oral medications that target specific immune pathways involved in eczema. Medications

like tofacitinib and baricitinib have shown promise in managing moderate to severe eczema, providing an alternative for individuals who may not respond to traditional treatments. Ongoing research is exploring their long-term safety and efficacy.

4. **Biologics**: Biologic medications, such as dupilumab, have revolutionized eczema treatment. Administered via injection, these drugs target specific proteins involved in the immune response. Dupilumab, for instance, inhibits interleukins associated with inflammation. Biologics are often prescribed for individuals with severe eczema who haven't responded well to other treatments. Regular monitoring is crucial, and the benefits and risks are carefully considered.

5. **Antihistamines**: Oral antihistamines are sometimes recommended to manage itching associated with eczema. While they don't directly address the underlying causes of eczema, antihistamines can provide relief from pruritus, contributing to improved quality of life.

The use of systemic medications for eczema is typically reserved for cases where other treatment options have proven insufficient or when the condition is severe and significantly impacts the individual's well-being. The decision to use systemic medications involves a careful consideration of the potential benefits and risks, with close monitoring by healthcare professionals to manage side effects and ensure optimal outcomes. These medications are often part of a broader, multidimensional treatment plan that may include topical treatments, moisturizers, and lifestyle modifications to comprehensively manage eczema.

Phototherapy

Phototherapy, also known as light therapy, is a therapeutic approach in the management of eczema that involves exposing the skin to ultraviolet (UV) light under controlled conditions. This treatment modality is particularly beneficial for certain types of eczema, offering relief from symptoms and promoting skin healing. Phototherapy is typically administered in a clinical setting, and various forms of light are utilized to address different aspects of eczema pathology.

1. **Ultraviolet B (UVB) Phototherapy:** UVB phototherapy is one of the most common forms of

light therapy for eczema. This treatment utilizes UVB rays, a specific range of ultraviolet light, to penetrate the skin and modulate immune responses. UVB phototherapy is effective in reducing inflammation, itching, and the proliferation of abnormal skin cells. Treatment sessions are usually conducted in a controlled environment, and the duration and intensity of UVB exposure are gradually increased based on individual response.

2. **Narrowband UVB Phototherapy:** Narrowband UVB is a more targeted form of UVB phototherapy that utilizes a narrower spectrum of UVB light. This focused approach is believed to be more effective in treating eczema while minimizing potential side effects. Narrowband UVB phototherapy has shown positive outcomes in improving symptoms and extending the duration of remission in individuals with moderate to severe eczema.

3. **UVA Phototherapy with Psoralen (PUVA):** PUVA involves combining exposure to UVA light with the administration of a photosensitizing medication called psoralen. Psoralen makes the skin more responsive to UVA light, enhancing its therapeutic effects. While PUVA has been historically used for various skin

conditions, including psoriasis, its role in eczema treatment is more limited due to potential side effects and safety concerns.

4. **UV-Free Phototherapy:** Advancements in technology have introduced UV-free phototherapy options, such as light-emitting diode (LED) devices. These devices emit specific wavelengths of light, often in the visible spectrum, without UV exposure. UV-free phototherapy is designed to minimize the potential risks associated with UV radiation while still providing therapeutic benefits. Research is ongoing to explore the effectiveness of UV-free options in eczema management.

5. **Mechanism of Action:** The exact mechanisms by which phototherapy benefits eczema are not fully understood, but several theories exist. UV light is known to modulate the immune system, reducing inflammation and suppressing abnormal immune responses associated with eczema. Additionally, exposure to UV light can enhance the production of vitamin D in the skin, which may contribute to its anti-inflammatory effects.

6. **Treatment Schedule and Duration:** Phototherapy is typically administered in a series of sessions scheduled over several weeks. The frequency and duration of treatment sessions depend on the individual's response, the type of phototherapy used, and the severity of eczema. Healthcare professionals carefully monitor progress and adjust the treatment plan accordingly.

7. **Considerations and Risks:** While phototherapy can be an effective treatment for eczema, it is not without risks. Prolonged exposure to UV radiation carries potential side effects, including skin aging, increased risk of skin cancer, and, in some cases, exacerbation of existing skin conditions. The decision to undergo phototherapy is made after a thorough evaluation of potential benefits and risks, and it is crucial to adhere to safety guidelines.

8. **Suitability for Different Types of Eczema:** Phototherapy is generally more effective for certain types of eczema, such as atopic dermatitis and chronic hand eczema. Its role in other forms of eczema, including contact dermatitis, may vary. The healthcare provider considers the specific type and characteristics of eczema before recommending phototherapy.

In conclusion, phototherapy represents a valuable and established treatment option for eczema, particularly for individuals with moderate to severe forms of the condition. The controlled exposure to UV light can help manage symptoms and improve the overall quality of life for those affected by eczema. As with any medical intervention, careful evaluation, monitoring, and adherence to safety protocols are essential to ensure optimal outcomes while minimizing potential risks.

CHAPTER FIVE

LIFESTYLE MODIFICATIONS

Lifestyle modifications play a crucial role in the holistic management of eczema, contributing to symptom control, prevention of flare-ups, and overall skin health. Adopting a skin-friendly lifestyle can complement medical treatments and enhance the well-being of individuals with eczema.

- **Clothing Choices:** Opting for loose-fitting, breathable fabrics like cotton can reduce friction and irritation on the skin. Avoiding rough or scratchy materials helps minimize skin trauma, especially during eczema flare-ups.

- **Temperature and Humidity:** Maintaining a comfortable indoor environment with stable temperatures and humidity levels is beneficial for eczema management. Extreme temperatures and dry air can exacerbate skin dryness and irritation.

- **Hydration**: Staying well-hydrated is essential for maintaining healthy skin. Drinking an adequate amount of water supports overall skin function and helps prevent excessive dryness.

- **Stress Management**: Stress can trigger or worsen eczema symptoms. Employing stress management techniques, such as mindfulness, meditation, or yoga, can contribute to symptom relief and overall well-being.

- **Regular Exercise:** Engaging in regular, moderate exercise supports overall health, including skin function. However, individuals with eczema should choose activities that minimize sweating and irritation, and they should shower promptly after exercise.

Skin care routine

Establishing a consistent and gentle skincare routine is paramount for individuals managing eczema. A well-designed routine helps maintain the skin's integrity, alleviate symptoms, and prevent flare-ups. Here's a guide to building an effective eczema-friendly skincare regimen:

- **Cleansing**: Choose a mild, fragrance-free cleanser designed for sensitive skin. Avoid harsh soaps or cleansers with strong detergents that can strip the skin of natural oils. Gentle cleansing helps remove impurities without exacerbating dryness or irritation.

- **Bathing Practices:** Take short, lukewarm baths or showers, as prolonged exposure to hot water can worsen eczema symptoms. Use soap sparingly and opt for non-soap cleansers or emollient washes. Pat the skin dry with a soft towel instead of rubbing to prevent friction.

- **Moisturization**: Moisturizing is a cornerstone of eczema management. Apply a hypoallergenic, fragrance-free moisturizer immediately after bathing and throughout the day as needed. Emollients help lock in moisture, soothe the skin, and strengthen the skin barrier.

- **Emollients and Ointments:** Select emollients or ointments over lotions, as they provide a thicker barrier and are more effective in preventing water loss from the skin. Petroleum-based ointments or products with ingredients like ceramides can be particularly beneficial for eczema-prone skin.

- **Avoiding Irritants:** Identify and avoid skincare products with potential irritants, such as fragrances, dyes, and alcohol. Opt for products labeled as hypoallergenic and suitable for sensitive skin to minimize the risk of triggering eczema flares.

- **Sun Protection**: Protecting the skin from the sun is crucial, as sun exposure can worsen eczema symptoms. Use a broad-spectrum sunscreen with at least SPF 30 when outdoors. Choose sunscreens designed for sensitive skin and free of potential allergens.

- **Clothing Choices:** Opt for loose-fitting, breathable clothing made from natural fabrics like cotton. Avoid wool and synthetic materials that may cause friction and irritation. Dressing in layers can help regulate body temperature without compromising the skin.

- **Avoiding Scratching:** Encourage gentle patting or tapping instead of scratching to alleviate itching. Keep nails short to reduce the risk of skin damage due to scratching. If scratching persists, consider using soft, breathable gloves during sleep.

- **Patch Testing:** Conduct patch testing when introducing new skincare products to identify potential allergens or irritants. Apply a small amount of the product on a small area of skin and monitor for any adverse reactions before widespread use.

A personalized skincare routine, tailored to individual needs and triggers, is crucial for effectively managing eczema. Regular communication with a healthcare professional ensures that the skincare regimen aligns with specific skin conditions and optimizes the overall management of eczematous symptoms.

Dietary considerations

Dietary considerations play a role in managing eczema, although the impact varies among individuals. While there is no one-size-fits-all diet for eczema, certain dietary factors may influence symptoms in some cases. Here are key considerations for individuals managing eczema:

- **Identifying Trigger Foods:** Some individuals with eczema may experience symptom flares related to specific foods. Common triggers include dairy, eggs, nuts, soy, wheat, and certain additives. Keeping a food diary and working with a healthcare professional or dietitian can help identify potential culprits.

- **Elimination Diets:** In cases where specific food triggers are suspected, elimination diets may be employed. This involves temporarily removing potential allergens from the diet and gradually reintroducing them while monitoring for eczema flares. Elimination diets should be conducted under the guidance of a healthcare professional to ensure proper nutrition.

- **Anti-Inflammatory Diets:** Incorporating anti-inflammatory foods into the diet may benefit some individuals with eczema. Foods rich in omega-3 fatty acids, such as fatty fish and flaxseeds, have anti-inflammatory properties. Antioxidant-rich fruits and vegetables also contribute to overall skin health.

- **Hydration**: Staying well-hydrated is essential for maintaining skin health. Drinking an adequate amount of water helps prevent dehydration, which can contribute to dry skin and exacerbate eczema symptoms.

- **Probiotics and Gut Health:** Some research suggests a link between gut health and eczema. Probiotics, found in fermented foods like yogurt or taken as supplements, may positively influence the gut microbiome. While evidence is evolving, incorporating probiotics into the diet may be considered under the guidance of a healthcare professional.

- **Individual Responses:** Dietary responses can vary widely among individuals with eczema. What works for one person may not be effective for another. It's essential to approach dietary changes with patience and to monitor the impact on eczema symptoms over time.

- **Consultation with Healthcare Professionals:** Before making significant dietary changes, individuals with eczema should consult with healthcare professionals, including allergists or dietitians. These experts can provide personalized guidance, conduct allergy testing if necessary, and ensure that dietary modifications align with overall health needs.

While dietary considerations may contribute to eczema management, it's crucial to emphasize that they are just one aspect of a comprehensive approach. Skincare practices, lifestyle modifications, and, when needed, medical interventions are equally important. Individuals should work collaboratively with healthcare professionals to create a well-rounded plan that addresses their specific triggers and symptoms

Allergen management

Effectively managing allergens is crucial for individuals with eczema, as exposure to specific triggers can contribute to flare-ups and exacerbate symptoms. Implementing allergen management strategies involves identifying potential allergens, minimizing exposure, and creating an environment that supports skin health. Here are key considerations for allergen management in eczema:

1. **Allergen Identification:** Work with healthcare professionals, such as allergists or dermatologists, to identify specific allergens that may trigger eczema flares. Allergy testing, including patch testing, can help pinpoint substances to which an individual may be sensitized.

2. **Skincare Product Selection:** Choose skincare products carefully, opting for those labeled as hypoallergenic and free of common irritants such as fragrances, dyes, and harsh chemicals. Patch testing new products before widespread use can help identify potential allergens in skincare routines.

3. **Environmental Allergens:** Minimize exposure to environmental allergens, such as pollen, dust mites, and pet dander. Regular cleaning, using allergen-proof bedding, and maintaining a clean and well-ventilated living space can contribute to allergen reduction.

4. **Clothing and Fabric Choices:** Select clothing made from natural, breathable fabrics like cotton. Avoid fabrics that may cause irritation, such as wool or synthetic materials. Wash new clothing before wearing to remove potential allergens from manufacturing processes.

5. **Allergen-Free Bedroom:** Create an allergen-free zone in the bedroom to promote better sleep and skin health. This may involve using hypoallergenic bedding, regularly washing sheets and pillowcases in hot water, and minimizing soft furnishings that can harbor dust mites.

6. **Dietary Considerations:** Identify and manage potential food allergens that may contribute to eczema symptoms. Consult with healthcare professionals or dietitians to conduct allergy testing or elimination diets to identify and eliminate trigger foods.

7. **Pet Allergens:** For individuals sensitive to pet dander, minimizing exposure to furry pets or creating pet-free zones in the home may be necessary. Regular grooming and cleaning can help reduce airborne pet allergens.

8. **Allergen Avoidance at Work or School:** Communicate with employers or school administrators about potential allergens in the workplace or educational environment. Implement strategies to reduce exposure, such as using allergen-proof covers for workspaces or classrooms.

9. **Regular Monitoring:** Regularly monitor and reassess allergen management strategies based on changes in symptoms and environmental factors. Adjustments may be necessary as seasons change, or new potential allergens are identified.

Creating an allergen-friendly environment is an ongoing process that requires vigilance and collaboration with healthcare professionals. Tailoring allergen management strategies to individual triggers and consistently implementing preventive measures can significantly contribute to the effective management of eczema and improve overall skin health.

CHAPTER SIX

COPING WITH ECZEMA

Coping with eczema involves a multifaceted approach that addresses both the physical and emotional aspects of living with this chronic skin condition.

Emotional and psychological impact

Living with eczema extends beyond physical symptoms, often influencing emotional and psychological well-being. The visible nature of skin conditions can contribute to a range of emotions, from self-consciousness to frustration. Understanding and addressing the emotional and psychological impact of eczema is crucial for comprehensive care.

- **Self-esteem and body image:** The visible manifestations of eczema, including redness, inflammation, and scarring, can affect self-esteem. Individuals may experience self-consciousness about their appearance, impacting body image and leading to feelings of embarrassment or inadequacy.

- **Anxiety and Depression:** Chronic conditions like eczema can contribute to heightened levels of anxiety and depression. The unpredictability of flare-ups, persistent symptoms, and the impact on daily life may generate feelings of uncertainty and distress.

- **Social Isolation:** Fear of judgment or discomfort due to visible skin conditions may lead to social withdrawal. Individuals with eczema might avoid social situations, impacting relationships and contributing to feelings of loneliness or isolation.

- **Impact on Daily Activities:** The practical challenges posed by eczema, such as discomfort, itching, and sleep disturbances, can influence daily activities. Concentration at work or school may suffer, impacting overall quality of life and productivity.

- **Impact on Children and Families:** Children with eczema may face unique challenges, with potential impacts on their social development and emotional well-being. Families may experience stress related to caregiving responsibilities and concerns about their child's quality of life.

- **Impact on Relationships:** Eczema can affect intimate relationships due to the emotional toll on individuals and the practical aspects of managing the condition. Open communication and mutual understanding are crucial for navigating these challenges.

- **Stigma and Misconceptions:** Stigma surrounding skin conditions can contribute to misconceptions about eczema. Individuals may encounter insensitive comments or judgment, adding to the emotional burden of managing their condition.

Support systems and resources

Support systems and resources play a crucial role in helping individuals cope with the challenges of living with eczema.

These networks provide emotional assistance, valuable information, and a sense of belonging, contributing to improved overall well-being. Here are key aspects of support systems and resources for individuals with eczema:

- **Healthcare Professionals:** Establishing a strong partnership with healthcare professionals, including dermatologists, allergists, and general practitioners, is essential. Regular check-ups and open communication ensure that individuals receive appropriate medical guidance, treatment adjustments, and ongoing support.

- **Patient Advocacy Organizations:** Patient advocacy organizations, such as the National Eczema Association (NEA) and local eczema support groups, offer a wealth of resources. These organizations provide information on the latest research, treatment options, and connect individuals with a community of others facing similar challenges.

- **Online Communities:** Virtual platforms, including online forums and social media groups, provide a space for individuals with eczema to share experiences, exchange advice, and offer emotional support. These communities foster a sense of understanding and solidarity, reducing feelings of isolation.

- **Educational Resources:** Access to reliable educational resources is vital for individuals and their caregivers. Educational materials from reputable sources, including healthcare providers and patient advocacy organizations, empower individuals with knowledge about eczema management, treatment options, and lifestyle modifications.

- **Mental Health Support:** Incorporating mental health professionals, such as psychologists or counselors, into the support network is crucial. Addressing the emotional impact of eczema through therapy or counseling helps individuals develop coping mechanisms and navigate the psychological challenges associated with the condition.

- **Family and Friends:** Building a support network that includes family and friends is invaluable. Their understanding, empathy, and encouragement contribute to emotional well-being and enhance the overall quality of life for individuals with eczema.

- **Skincare Experts:** Collaborating with skincare professionals, such as estheticians or skincare specialists, can provide practical tips for managing eczema symptoms. These experts can offer guidance on suitable skincare products and routines tailored to individual needs.

- **Telehealth Services:** Telehealth services offer convenient access to healthcare professionals, especially for individuals who may face challenges with in-person visits. Virtual consultations provide ongoing support and guidance, contributing to effective eczema management.

- **Work and School Support:** Individuals with eczema may benefit from workplace or school accommodations to manage their condition effectively. Open communication with employers, teachers, and colleagues fosters understanding and support.

- **Holistic Wellness Practices:** Exploring holistic wellness practices, such as yoga, meditation, or stress-reduction techniques, can complement medical treatments. Integrating these practices into daily life supports emotional and mental well-being.

Support systems and resources for eczema extend beyond the medical realm, encompassing emotional, informational, and practical assistance. By actively engaging with these networks, individuals with eczema can enhance their ability to cope with the condition, improve their quality of life, and foster a more comprehensive approach to managing eczema.

Importance of mental health support

The importance of mental health support for individuals with eczema cannot be overstated, as the condition's impact extends beyond the physical realm to influence emotional well-being. Here are key reasons highlighting the significance of mental health support in eczema management:

◆ **Emotional Toll of Visible Symptoms:** Eczema's visible symptoms, including redness, inflammation, and scarring, can lead to emotional distress. Individuals may experience feelings of self-consciousness, embarrassment, or frustration, emphasizing the need for mental health support to address these emotional challenges.

◆ **Anxiety and Depression Management:** Living with a chronic condition like eczema can contribute to heightened levels of anxiety and depression. Mental health support provides individuals with tools and coping strategies to manage these mental health challenges effectively.

- **Stress Reduction:** Stress is a known trigger for eczema flares, creating a cyclical relationship between the condition and mental well-being. Mental health support helps individuals identify and manage stressors, reducing the likelihood of exacerbating eczema symptoms.

- **Coping Mechanisms and Resilience:** Coping with the chronic nature of eczema requires resilience. Mental health professionals can assist individuals in developing adaptive coping mechanisms, fostering emotional strength to navigate the challenges associated with the condition.

- **Support for Families and Caregivers:** Mental health support extends beyond individuals with eczema to their families and caregivers. Coping with the demands of caregiving, understanding the emotional impact on their loved ones, and seeking guidance on providing effective support are crucial aspects addressed through mental health support.

- **Improved Quality of Life:** Addressing the mental health aspects of eczema contributes to an overall improved quality of life. Individuals who receive adequate mental health support often report better emotional well-being, increased self-esteem, and a more positive outlook on managing their condition.

◆ **Open Communication and Expression:** Mental health support provides a safe space for individuals to express their emotions, fears, and challenges related to eczema. Open communication with mental health professionals fosters a deeper understanding of the psychological impact and allows for tailored interventions.

◆ **Integrated Healthcare Approach:** A holistic approach to eczema management acknowledges the interconnectedness of physical and mental health. Integrated care, combining dermatological treatment with mental health support, ensures a comprehensive approach to addressing the challenges associated with eczema.

◆ **Personalized Strategies for Coping:** Every individual's experience with eczema is unique. Mental health support allows for the development of personalized strategies for coping, considering individual triggers, lifestyle factors, and emotional responses to the condition.

In conclusion, mental health support is an integral component of eczema management. By addressing the emotional and psychological aspects of living with this chronic skin condition, individuals can develop resilience, manage stress, and ultimately enhance their ability to navigate the challenges of eczema in a holistic and empowering manner.

CHAPTER SEVEN

PREVENTION

Preventing eczema flare-ups involves a combination of lifestyle modifications, skincare practices, and environmental management. While eczema is a chronic condition, proactive measures can significantly reduce the frequency and severity of symptoms. Here's a comprehensive guide to eczema prevention

* **Skincare Routine:** Establishing a gentle and consistent skincare routine is foundational in preventing eczema flare-ups. Use mild, fragrance-free cleansers, and opt for emollient-rich moisturizers to keep the skin hydrated. Regular moisturization helps maintain the skin barrier, reducing the risk of irritants triggering flare-ups.

*

* **Avoiding Irritants:** Identify and avoid potential irritants that can trigger eczema symptoms. This includes harsh

soaps, fragrances, and certain fabrics. Choose hypoallergenic and fragrance-free products for skincare, laundry, and household cleaning to minimize the risk of skin irritation.

* **Moisture Maintenance:** Maintaining adequate skin moisture is crucial in preventing eczema. Take short, lukewarm baths or showers, and pat the skin dry gently. Apply moisturizer immediately after bathing to lock in moisture. In drier climates, using a humidifier in living spaces can help combat dry air.

* **Clothing Choices:** Select soft, breathable fabrics like cotton to minimize friction and irritation. Avoid tight clothing, and consider wearing layers that allow better temperature regulation without causing discomfort to the skin.

* **Allergen Management:** Identify and manage allergens that may trigger eczema flares. This may involve allergy testing to determine specific sensitivities. Once identified, take steps to minimize exposure to these allergens, whether they are in skincare products, the environment, or certain foods.

* **Temperature and Humidity Control:** Maintain a comfortable indoor environment by controlling temperature and humidity levels. Extreme temperatures and low humidity can contribute to skin dryness and irritation. Dress appropriately for weather conditions, and consider using a humidifier in dry environments.

* **Stress Management:** Stress is a known trigger for eczema flare-ups. Incorporate stress management techniques into daily life, such as mindfulness, meditation, or yoga. Regular exercise and engaging in relaxing activities contribute to overall stress reduction.

* **Diet and Hydration:** While the direct impact of diet on eczema varies among individuals, staying hydrated and maintaining a balanced diet can support skin health. Identify and manage any specific food triggers through consultation with healthcare professionals or dietitians.

* **Avoiding Scratching:** Scratching can exacerbate eczema symptoms and lead to further skin damage. Encourage gentle patting or tapping instead of scratching to relieve itching. Keeping nails short and using soft gloves during sleep can prevent unintentional scratching.

- ❖ **Sun Protection:** Protect the skin from the sun by using broad-spectrum sunscreen with at least SPF 30. Sun exposure can worsen eczema symptoms, so sun protection is crucial, especially during outdoor activities.

- ❖ **Regular Check-ups:** Schedule regular check-ups with healthcare professionals to monitor eczema management and make necessary adjustments to treatment plans. Discuss any changes in symptoms, triggers, or lifestyle that may impact eczema prevention.

- ❖ **Allergy-proofing Living Spaces:** Minimize potential allergens in living spaces by using allergen-proof covers for pillows and mattresses, regularly cleaning and dusting, and keeping pet dander under control if applicable.

- ❖ **Clothing and Bedding Care:** Wash clothing and bedding in hypoallergenic and fragrance-free detergents. Rinse items thoroughly to remove any remaining detergent residues that may irritate the skin.

Early intervention strategies

Early intervention is crucial in managing eczema effectively and preventing the escalation of symptoms. Implementing timely strategies helps address flare-ups, soothe irritated skin, and minimize the impact of the condition. Here are key early intervention strategies for eczema management:

- ❖ **Prompt Skincare:** At the first sign of eczema symptoms, initiate a gentle and consistent skincare routine. Use mild, fragrance-free cleansers, and apply moisturizers immediately after bathing to lock in moisture. Early moisturization helps alleviate dryness and supports the skin barrier.

- ❖ **Topical Treatments:** For localized flare-ups, consider applying over-the-counter or prescribed topical treatments. These may include corticosteroid creams or ointments, calcineurin inhibitors, or other anti-inflammatory agents. Consult with healthcare professionals to determine the most suitable option based on the severity and location of symptoms.

- ❖ **Avoiding Triggers:** Identify and eliminate potential triggers promptly. Whether allergens in skincare products, environmental factors, or certain foods, understanding and avoiding triggers at the early stages can prevent symptom exacerbation.

❖ **Cool Compresses:** Apply cool compresses to areas experiencing inflammation and itching. This can provide immediate relief by reducing redness and soothing irritated skin. Avoid hot water or harsh ice packs, as extreme temperatures can worsen eczema symptoms.

❖ **Anti-Itch Solutions:** Utilize over-the-counter anti-itch creams or ointments containing ingredients like colloidal oatmeal or menthol. These can help alleviate itching and provide comfort during flare-ups. It's essential to choose products that are compatible with sensitive skin.

❖ **Allergen Management:** Promptly address exposure to allergens by adjusting skincare products, household items, or dietary choices. Identifying and managing allergens early on contributes to minimizing the risk of recurrent flare-ups.

❖ **Consult Healthcare Professionals:** If symptoms persist or worsen despite initial interventions, seek prompt guidance from healthcare professionals. Dermatologists or general practitioners can assess the situation, adjust treatment plans, or recommend additional interventions based on individual needs.

❖ **Re-evaluation of Treatment Plans:** Regularly reevaluate and adjust treatment plans based on the evolving nature of eczema symptoms. This may involve modifying skincare routines, updating medication prescriptions, or exploring new therapeutic approaches to better manage the condition.

By implementing these early intervention strategies, individuals with eczema can actively manage symptoms, enhance their quality of life, and minimize the impact of the condition. Timely attention to eczema symptoms sets the stage for effective long-term management and prevention of recurrent flare-ups.

CHAPTER EIGHTH

SPECIAL CONSIDERATIONS

Special considerations in eczema management involve tailoring approaches to unique situations. For infants and children, gentle skincare practices, allergen identification, and close pediatric supervision are crucial. Pregnancy may require adjustments to treatment plans, considering both maternal and fetal well-being. Individuals with comorbid conditions, like asthma or allergies, may need integrated care. Ethnic variations and cultural factors can influence skincare practices.

Eczema in children

Eczema in children, often referred to as atopic dermatitis, is a common and chronic skin condition that requires special attention and care. Recognizing and managing eczema in children involves a combination of skincare practices, allergen identification, and ongoing support.

- **Gentle Skincare:** Children's skin is delicate, and a gentle skincare routine is paramount. Use mild, fragrance-free cleansers and moisturizers to prevent skin dryness. Regular moisturization helps maintain the skin barrier, reducing the likelihood of eczema flare-ups.

- **Allergen Identification:** Identifying and managing allergens is crucial in pediatric eczema. Conducting allergy testing can help pinpoint triggers, whether they are related to specific foods, environmental factors, or skincare products. Avoiding these allergens plays a key role in preventing flare-ups.

- **Avoiding Irritants:** Children's skin is more sensitive to irritants, so it's essential to choose hypoallergenic and fragrance-free products. This includes laundry detergents, soaps, and clothing materials. Minimizing exposure to potential irritants helps maintain skin health.

- **Monitoring Scratching:** Children may find it challenging to resist scratching, which can exacerbate eczema symptoms. Keep children's nails short, and consider using soft mittens or gloves during sleep to prevent unintentional scratching.

- **Pediatric Supervision:** Regular check-ups with pediatricians or dermatologists are vital for monitoring the child's skin health. Healthcare professionals can guide parents on appropriate skincare routines, recommend suitable treatments, and adjust management plans based on the child's unique needs.

- **Dietary Considerations:** Identifying and managing food allergens is crucial in pediatric eczema. Working with healthcare professionals, including allergists and dietitians, can help determine if specific foods contribute to eczema flare-ups, leading to dietary adjustments when necessary.

- **Emotional Support:** Eczema can impact a child's emotional well-being. Provide emotional support, and encourage open communication about how the child feels regarding their skin condition. Creating a supportive environment fosters resilience and helps children cope with the challenges of living with eczema.

- **Lifestyle Modifications:** Implementing lifestyle modifications, such as choosing breathable fabrics, maintaining a comfortable indoor environment, and managing stressors, contributes to overall pediatric eczema management.

In summary, managing eczema in children requires a comprehensive and attentive approach. By focusing on gentle skincare, allergen identification, pediatric supervision, and emotional support, parents and caregivers can effectively navigate the challenges associated with pediatric eczema and promote healthy skin development in their children.

Eczema in pregnancy

Eczema during pregnancy, also known as gestational eczema, can present unique challenges for expectant mothers. Hormonal changes, immune system variations, and stress can influence eczema symptoms during this time. Here are considerations and strategies for managing eczema during pregnancy:

- **Hormonal Impact:** Pregnancy hormones, particularly estrogen and progesterone, can influence eczema symptoms. While some women experience improvement, others may notice exacerbation of symptoms. This variability highlights the importance of personalized care and monitoring.

- **Skincare Adjustments:** Adapting skincare routines is crucial during pregnancy. Opt for fragrance-free, hypoallergenic products to minimize the risk of skin irritation. Regular moisturization helps maintain skin hydration, reducing the likelihood of eczema flare-ups.

- **Consultation with Healthcare Professionals:** Expectant mothers should consult with healthcare professionals, including dermatologists and obstetricians, to discuss eczema management during pregnancy. Certain medications commonly used for eczema may need to be adjusted or avoided during this period, necessitating careful evaluation and guidance.

- **Avoiding Triggers:** Identifying and avoiding triggers become especially important during pregnancy. Stress management, maintaining a comfortable environment, and minimizing exposure to potential allergens contribute to preventing eczema exacerbation.

- **Dietary Considerations:** Pregnant women with eczema may explore dietary considerations under the guidance of healthcare professionals. While there's limited evidence linking specific foods to eczema, some individuals may find that certain dietary adjustments positively impact their skin health.

- **Clothing Choices:** Selecting loose-fitting, breathable clothing can help prevent skin irritation. Cotton fabrics are gentle on the skin and reduce friction, promoting comfort for pregnant women with eczema.

- **Emotional Well-being:** Pregnancy itself can be emotionally demanding, and managing eczema during this time requires attention to emotional well-being. Stress is a known trigger for eczema flare-ups, so adopting stress-reduction techniques such as mindfulness, relaxation exercises, or prenatal yoga can be beneficial.

- **Medication Considerations:** Discussing medication options with healthcare providers is crucial during pregnancy. While some topical treatments are generally considered safe, certain systemic medications may need to be adjusted or avoided. Open communication with healthcare professionals ensures that the chosen treatment plan aligns with the well-being of both the mother and the developing fetus.

- **Monitoring Skin Changes:** Expectant mothers should closely monitor changes in their skin throughout pregnancy. Any unusual or persistent symptoms should be promptly discussed with healthcare providers to address potential issues early.

- **Postpartum Considerations:** Eczema management may continue to evolve postpartum. Hormonal changes, breastfeeding considerations, and the demands of caring for a newborn can impact eczema symptoms. Regular follow-ups with healthcare professionals help adjust strategies as needed.

- **Breastfeeding Considerations:** If breastfeeding, mothers should be cautious about potential irritants in skincare products that may come into contact with the baby's skin. Discussing suitable products with healthcare providers ensures the safety of both mother and child.

In conclusion, managing eczema during pregnancy involves a combination of skincare adjustments, consultation with healthcare professionals, and attention to emotional well-being. Every woman's experience is unique, and individualized care is essential. By actively addressing the specific challenges associated with eczema during pregnancy, expectant mothers can navigate this period with optimal skin health and overall well-being.

CHAPTER 9

RESEARCH AND INNOVATIONS

Ongoing research and innovations in eczema aim to enhance understanding, treatment options, and overall quality of life for individuals with the condition. Studies explore new therapies, skincare technologies, and personalized approaches. Innovations include advanced topical treatments, targeted immunotherapies, and precision medicine based on genetic insights. As research progresses, a more comprehensive understanding of eczema's underlying mechanisms emerges, fostering continuous advancements in medical and skincare strategies to better manage and improve the lives of those affected by eczema.

Ongoing research

> **Immunotherapy and Biologics:** Research is exploring the use of immunotherapies and biologics to target specific immune responses associated with eczema. These innovative treatments aim to modulate the immune system, providing more targeted and effective management of eczema symptoms.

> **Precision Medicine:** Advancements in genetics are contributing to the development of precision medicine for eczema. Researchers are investigating genetic factors that may influence an individual's susceptibility to eczema, allowing for tailored treatment plans based on a person's unique genetic profile.

> **Barrier Repair Therapies:** Understanding the importance of the skin barrier in eczema, research focuses on developing barrier repair therapies. These interventions aim to enhance the skin's natural protective mechanisms, reducing susceptibility to irritants and preventing flare-ups.

➢ **Microbiome Research:** The skin's microbiome, the community of microorganisms living on the skin, plays a role in eczema. Ongoing research explores the connection between the skin microbiome and eczema, offering insights into potential microbiome-targeted therapies for symptom management.

➢ **Environmental Triggers:** Researchers are investigating environmental factors that may trigger or exacerbate eczema. This includes studying the impact of pollutants, climate conditions, and lifestyle factors, with the goal of identifying modifiable environmental elements to reduce the risk of flare-ups.

➢ **Patient-Reported Outcomes:** To better understand the impact of eczema on individuals' lives, research incorporates patient-reported outcomes. Studying the physical and emotional burden of eczema helps guide the development of treatments that align with patients' needs and priorities.

➢ **Telemedicine and Digital Health Solutions:** Advancements in telemedicine and digital health solutions offer innovative ways to monitor and manage eczema remotely. Mobile apps and wearable devices enable real-time tracking of symptoms, facilitating more personalized and accessible care.

➢ **Lifestyle Interventions:** Research emphasizes lifestyle interventions as a complementary approach to eczema management. Studies explore the impact of diet, stress reduction techniques, and behavioral modifications in reducing the frequency and severity of flare-ups.

By pushing the boundaries of scientific inquiry, ongoing research in eczema holds the promise of transforming the landscape of diagnosis and treatment. These developments not only enhance medical interventions but also empower individuals with eczema to actively participate in managing their condition through personalized and holistic approaches.

Emerging treatment and therapy

Emerging treatments and therapies in the field of eczema hold promise for revolutionizing the management of this chronic skin condition. Researchers and clinicians are exploring innovative approaches that aim to provide more targeted, effective, and personalized care. Here are some notable areas of development:

- **Topical Janus Kinase (JAK) Inhibitors:** JAK inhibitors, traditionally used in systemic treatments, are now being explored in topical formulations for eczema. These inhibitors target specific immune pathways involved in eczema inflammation, potentially offering a more localized and precise treatment option with fewer systemic side effects.

- **Dupilumab and Beyond:** Dupilumab, an FDA-approved biologic, has shown remarkable efficacy in treating moderate to severe eczema. Ongoing research is focused on developing similar biologics and exploring additional pathways for targeted therapies that can address specific immune responses associated with eczema.

- **Gene Therapy:** Advancements in gene therapy hold potential for treating eczema by addressing underlying genetic factors. Research is exploring ways to modify genes related to skin barrier function and immune response to develop targeted interventions tailored to an individual's genetic makeup.

- **Microbiome Modulation:** The skin microbiome, composed of various microorganisms, plays a role in eczema development. Emerging therapies aim to modulate the skin microbiome to restore a healthy balance, potentially reducing inflammation and preventing flare-ups.

✧ **CRISPR Technology:** The revolutionary CRISPR-Cas9 gene-editing technology is being investigated for its potential in addressing genetic factors linked to eczema. While still in the early stages, CRISPR offers the possibility of precise genetic modifications to correct underlying issues associated with the condition.

✧ **Small Molecule Therapies:** Researchers are exploring small molecule therapies that can be delivered topically or systemically to modulate specific pathways involved in eczema inflammation. These molecules target key proteins and signaling pathways, providing a novel approach to managing symptoms.

✧ **Digital Health Interventions:** In the realm of eczema management, digital health solutions are gaining prominence. Mobile apps and wearable devices offer real-time monitoring, providing insights into triggers and symptoms. These technologies facilitate more personalized and patient-centric approaches to care.

As these emerging treatments and therapies progress through clinical trials and research phases, they offer hope for a future where eczema management is not only more effective but also tailored to the individual characteristics of each patient. By targeting specific pathways, genetic factors, and the skin microbiome, these innovations aim to transform the landscape of eczema care, providing new avenues for improved quality of life for those affected by this challenging skin condition.

CHAPTER TEN

● PERSONAL STORIES AND

EXPERIENCES

Personal stories and experiences play a crucial role in understanding the impact of eczema beyond medical textbooks. Individuals affected by eczema often share their journeys, shedding light on the challenges, triumphs, and emotional aspects of living with this chronic skin condition.

- **Shared Understanding:** Personal stories create a shared understanding of eczema's diverse manifestations. Whether detailing the frustration of constant itching, the emotional toll of visible skin symptoms, or the journey to finding effective treatments, these narratives foster empathy and connection among individuals experiencing similar challenges.

- **Coping Strategies:** Listening to personal experiences provides insights into various coping strategies. From skincare routines and dietary modifications to mental health practices, individuals share what has worked for them. These firsthand accounts become valuable resources for others seeking practical advice in managing their eczema.

- **Encouragement and Support:** Sharing personal stories can be a source of encouragement and support for those feeling isolated in their eczema journey. Knowing that others have faced similar struggles and have found ways to navigate them can instill hope and resilience in individuals dealing with the condition.

- **Raising Awareness:** Personal stories contribute to raising awareness about the impact of eczema. They dispel myths, challenge misconceptions, and provide a human perspective that goes beyond clinical descriptions. This awareness is crucial for fostering understanding among the broader community.

- **Advocacy and Empowerment:** Many individuals with eczema become advocates for the condition, using their stories to raise awareness, promote research, and advocate for improved access to treatments. Personal experiences become powerful tools for empowering the eczema community and influencing positive change.

- **Highlighting Diversity:** Eczema manifests differently in each person, and personal stories highlight this diversity. From infants to adults, the experiences of individuals across different ages, backgrounds, and lifestyles contribute to a more nuanced understanding of eczema's impact on diverse populations.

- **Lessons Learned:** Personal stories often carry valuable lessons learned throughout the eczema journey. Individuals share insights into what they wish they had known earlier, what proved most effective, and how they adapted their lifestyles. These lessons become a guide for others entering their own eczema management path.

In essence, personal stories and experiences weave a tapestry of resilience, courage, and shared humanity within the eczema community. Whether shared through blogs, support groups, or advocacy platforms, these narratives empower individuals, raise awareness, and contribute to a more compassionate understanding of eczema's multifaceted impact on lives.

Insights from Caregivers

Insights from caregivers provide a unique and essential perspective on the challenges and responsibilities involved in supporting individuals with eczema. Caregivers, often family members or close friends, contribute valuable insights into the emotional, practical, and interpersonal dimensions of eczema management.

* **Emotional Impact:** Caregivers offer profound insights into the emotional impact of eczema on both the individual with the condition and themselves. Witnessing a loved one grapple with visible symptoms, discomfort, and emotional distress can be emotionally challenging. Caregivers share experiences of empathy, frustration, and the importance of fostering emotional resilience in both the patient and themselves.

* **Practical Support:** Caregivers play a crucial role in providing practical support for daily eczema

management. Their insights often include strategies for creating a supportive living environment, managing skincare routines, and adapting lifestyle factors to minimize triggers. These practical insights showcase the dedication and resourcefulness required in caring for someone with eczema.

❖ **Advocacy and Education:** Caregivers become advocates for individuals with eczema, actively seeking information, participating in healthcare decisions, and promoting awareness within their communities. Their insights contribute to the broader understanding of eczema's impact on families and drive advocacy efforts for improved access to treatments and support services.

❖ **Coping Strategies:** Understanding the unique challenges faced by caregivers, such as balancing caregiving responsibilities with their own well-being, is crucial. Insights from caregivers often include coping strategies, emphasizing the importance of self-care, seeking emotional support, and finding a balance between caregiving duties and personal needs.

❖ **Impact on Family Dynamics:** Caregiver narratives shed light on how eczema influences family dynamics. Siblings, parents, and extended family members may need to adapt to the demands of eczema care. These insights contribute to a holistic understanding of the condition's ripple effects within a family unit.

❖ **Shared Learning:** Caregiver insights serve as a source of shared learning within the caregiving community. Learning from others who have navigated similar challenges helps caregivers refine their approaches, discover new strategies, and build a supportive network.

In essence, insights from caregivers enrich the narrative surrounding eczema by offering a compassionate and comprehensive view of the condition's impact on individuals and their support systems. These narratives foster empathy, provide practical guidance, and contribute to the collective wisdom that strengthens the caregiving community for those affected by eczema.

CHAPTER 11

GLOSSARY

Key terms and definitions

This offers a comprehensive understanding of the condition, its management, and associated concepts

Eczema (Dermatitis):
Eczema is a chronic inflammatory skin condition characterized by red, itchy, and inflamed skin. It encompasses various types, with atopic dermatitis being the most common.
Atopic Dermatitis (AD):
Definition: Atopic dermatitis is a chronic and inflammatory form of eczema that often starts in infancy. It is associated

with a hypersensitive immune response, genetic factors, and a compromised skin barrier.

Contact Dermatitis:

Definition: Contact dermatitis is eczema triggered by direct skin contact with irritants or allergens. It can be categorized as irritant contact dermatitis (non-allergic) or allergic contact dermatitis (immune response).

Seborrheic Dermatitis:

Definition: Seborrheic dermatitis is a form of eczema that primarily affects areas rich in oil glands, such as the scalp, face, and upper chest. It is characterized by red, scaly patches.

Stasis Dermatitis:

Stasis dermatitis occurs due to poor circulation, often in the lower legs. It results in skin inflammation and is commonly associated with venous insufficiency.

Nummular Dermatitis:

Nummular dermatitis presents as coin-shaped lesions on the skin. It is often triggered by skin dryness and may be more prevalent in winter.

Pruritus:

Pruritus refers to intense itching of the skin, a common symptom in eczema. It can lead to scratching, potentially exacerbating the condition.

Skin Barrier:
The skin barrier is the outermost layer of the skin that acts as a protective shield. In eczema, the skin barrier is compromised, leading to increased vulnerability to irritants and allergens.

Topical Corticosteroids:
Topical corticosteroids are anti-inflammatory medications applied directly to the skin. They are a common treatment for eczema to reduce inflammation and itching.

Emollients/Moisturizers:
Emollients or moisturizers are substances that hydrate and soften the skin. Regular use helps in maintaining the skin barrier and preventing dryness in eczema.

Flare-up:
A flare-up refers to a sudden and intense episode of worsening eczema symptoms, characterized by increased redness, itching, and inflammation.

Triggers:

Triggers are factors that can exacerbate eczema symptoms. Common triggers include certain foods, allergens, stress, and environmental factors.

Allergen:
An allergen is a substance that can trigger an allergic reaction. In eczema, allergens may contribute to skin inflammation.

Patch Testing:
Patch testing is a diagnostic procedure used to identify allergens causing contact dermatitis. Small amounts of potential allergens are applied to the skin to observe reactions.

Immunotherapy:
Immunotherapy involves desensitizing the immune system to allergens. It is not commonly used for eczema but may be considered in specific cases.

Antihistamines:
Antihistamines are medications that block histamine receptors, helping to alleviate itching in eczema and other allergic conditions.

Dupilumab:

Dupilumab is a biologic medication used to treat moderate to severe atopic dermatitis. It inhibits specific immune pathways involved in eczema.

Phototherapy:
Phototherapy involves exposing the skin to ultraviolet (UV) light under controlled conditions. It can be an effective treatment for certain types of eczema.

Systemic Medications:
Systemic medications are taken orally or injected to treat eczema. They may include immunosuppressants or other medications that affect the entire body.

Colloidal Oatmeal:
Colloidal oatmeal is finely ground oats suspended in liquid. It is used in skincare products to relieve itching and soothe inflamed skin in eczema.

Wet Wrap Therapy:
Wet wrap therapy involves applying emollients to the skin and covering with wet bandages. It helps hydrate the skin and reduce inflammation.

Hypoallergenic:

Hypoallergenic products are designed to minimize the risk of causing allergic reactions. They are commonly recommended for individuals with sensitive skin, including those with eczema.

Asteatotic Eczema:
Asteatotic eczema, also known as xerotic eczema, is characterized by dry, cracked, and fissured skin. It is often associated with aging and dry environments.

Eczema Herpeticum:
Eczema herpeticum is a rare but serious complication where the herpes simplex virus infects eczema-affected skin, leading to widespread infection.

Corticosteroid Withdrawal:
Corticosteroid withdrawal refers to the rebound worsening of eczema symptoms upon discontinuing topical corticosteroids after prolonged use.

Diluted Bleach Baths:
Diluted bleach baths involve adding a small amount of bleach to bathwater. It is used as a preventive measure to reduce the risk of bacterial skin infections in eczema.

Eczema Action Plan:

An eczema action plan is a personalized guide outlining steps to manage and prevent eczema flare-ups. It includes skincare routines, triggers to avoid, and emergency measures.

Filaggrin:

Filaggrin is a protein crucial for maintaining the skin barrier. Genetic mutations affecting filaggrin are associated with an increased risk of eczema.

Microbiome:

The skin microbiome refers to the community of microorganisms living on the skin. Maintaining a healthy microbiome is important for skin health in eczema.

Lichenification:

Lichenification is the thickening and hardening of the skin due to chronic scratching or rubbing, commonly seen in long-standing eczema.

TCS (Topical Corticosteroid) Potency:

TCS potency refers to the strength or concentration of topical corticosteroid medications. Potency levels range from mild to very potent, influencing their effectiveness and potential side effects.

Eczema Registry:

An eczema registry is a database that collects and analyzes information on individuals with eczema. It aids in research, treatment development, and understanding the condition's epidemiology.

Treatments of Last Resort:

Treatments of last resort are interventions considered when other therapeutic options have failed. They may include systemic medications with significant side effects and risks.

Emotional Well-being:

Emotional well-being refers to the psychological and emotional state of an individual. Addressing emotional well-being is essential in the holistic management of eczema.

Patient-Centered Care:

Patient-centered care emphasizes involving patients in healthcare decisions, tailoring treatment plans to individual needs, and considering patients' preferences and values.

Ceramides:

Ceramides are lipid molecules naturally present in the skin's outer layer. Skincare products containing ceramides help enhance the skin barrier in eczema.

Biopsy:
A biopsy involves taking a small sample of skin for examination under a microscope. It may be done to diagnose certain types of eczema or rule out other skin conditions.

Eczema Clothing:
Eczema clothing is designed to minimize skin irritation. It is often made from soft, breathable fabrics without irritating seams or tags.

Dietary Elimination:
Dietary elimination involves removing specific foods from the diet to identify and manage potential triggers contributing to eczema symptoms.

Hydrocortisone:
Hydrocortisone is a mild topical corticosteroid available over-the-counter. It is commonly used for mild eczema symptoms.

Autoimmune Diseases:
Autoimmune diseases involve the immune system mistakenly attacking the body's own tissues. While eczema is not

autoimmune, it shares immune system involvement with some autoimmune conditions.

Psychodermatology:

Psychodermatology is a field that explores the relationship between psychological factors and skin conditions, including eczema. It emphasizes a holistic approach to treatment.

Eczema Vaccination Guidelines:

Eczema vaccination guidelines provide recommendations for individuals with eczema regarding vaccinations. Some precautions may be necessary to prevent adverse reactions.

Barrier Repair Therapies:

Barrier repair therapies aim to enhance the skin barrier function. They include emollients, moisturizers, and products containing lipids to support skin health in eczema.

Mental Health Support:

Mental health support involves addressing psychological well-being in eczema management. It may include counseling, therapy, and stress management strategies.

Tape Stripping:

Tape stripping is a research technique involving applying and removing adhesive tape to the skin. It is used to collect samples for studying the skin barrier in eczema.

Eczema Gloves and Wraps:
Eczema gloves and wraps are designed to cover and protect the hands or affected areas. They are often made from soft materials to prevent scratching.

Placebo Effect:
The placebo effect refers to the perceived improvement in symptoms due to the psychological belief in the effectiveness of a treatment, even if it has no therapeutic value.

Skin pH:
Skin pH refers to the acidity or alkalinity of the skin. Maintaining the appropriate pH is crucial for skin barrier function and overall skin health in eczema.

Eczema Education:
Eczema education involves providing information and resources to individuals, caregivers, and healthcare professionals to enhance understanding and management of eczema.

This extensive list of key terms and definitions aims to empower readers with a comprehensive understanding of eczema, from its clinical manifestations to various treatment modalities and associated concepts.

Chapter 12

Resources

Recommend reading materials

Recommended reading materials can be valuable companions for individuals seeking in-depth knowledge about eczema, its management, and related topics. Here are some highly recommended books for comprehensive insights:

The Eczema Diet: Eczema-safe food to stop the itch and prevent eczema for life, by Karen Fischer:
This book delves into the connection between diet and eczema, offering practical advice on eczema-safe foods and lifestyle changes.

Eczema: The Definitive Eczema Cure - How To Overcome Eczema Forever And Live Your Life!, by Michael Adams:
Michael Adams provides insights into overcoming eczema by addressing its root causes, offering guidance on treatments and lifestyle changes.

Eczema Healing: A Comprehensive Guide to a Healthy Gut and Skin, by Rebecca Bonneteau:
Rebecca Bonneteau explores the gut-skin connection, emphasizing the role of a healthy gut in managing eczema and promoting overall skin wellness.

The Eczema Solution, by Sue Armstrong-Brown:
Sue Armstrong-Brown shares her personal journey with eczema and provides practical advice on managing the condition through skincare, diet, and stress reduction.

Eczema: The 'At Your Fingertips' Guide, by Tim Mitchell and Márta Telek:

A comprehensive guide that covers various aspects of eczema, from understanding the condition to available treatments and self-care strategies.

The Eczema Detox: The Low-Chemical Diet for Eliminating Skin Inflammation, by Karen Fischer:

Karen Fischer introduces a low-chemical diet to help eliminate skin inflammation and manage eczema symptoms.

The Eczema Solution, by Sue Armstrong-Brown:

This book combines personal experiences with practical advice, offering a holistic approach to eczema management, including skincare, diet, and lifestyle adjustments.

Eczema-Free for Life, by Adnan Nasir:

Dr. Adnan Nasir provides a comprehensive guide to understanding eczema triggers, effective treatments, and long-term strategies for managing and preventing flare-ups.

The Complete Guide to Eczema and Psoriasis, by Leopoldo Ferriera:

Dr. Leopoldo Ferriera offers a thorough guide covering eczema and psoriasis, including their causes, symptoms, and evidence-based treatments.

Living with Eczema: Mom Asks, Doc Answers!, by Amy Brodsky, MD, and Christine Clark, MD:

Written by dermatologists, this book addresses common questions and concerns about eczema, providing expert insights and guidance.

These recommended readings cater to various preferences, whether you're looking for practical advice, personal narratives, or a scientific understanding of eczema. They empower individuals to make informed decisions about their health and well-being while navigating the complexities of eczema.

Support Organizations

Support organizations play a crucial role in offering assistance, guidance, and a sense of community for individuals affected by eczema. These organizations are dedicated to providing resources, support networks, and advocacy efforts to enhance the well-being of those dealing with this chronic skin condition. Here are notable support organizations making a difference:

National Eczema Association (NEA):
The NEA is a leading organization committed to improving the lives of individuals with eczema. They provide educational resources, support groups, and advocacy

initiatives. Their website offers a wealth of information on eczema management, treatment options, and community forums for sharing experiences.

Eczema Society of Canada:

The Eczema Society of Canada focuses on raising awareness, offering support, and providing educational resources for individuals and families affected by eczema. They organize events, share research updates, and connect individuals with eczema-related information.

Eczema Outreach Support (EOS):

Based in the United Kingdom, EOS offers support to families and individuals dealing with eczema. They provide practical advice, organize events, and facilitate a supportive community through online forums and local meet-ups.

Eczema Association Australasia (EAA):

Serving the Australasia region, the EAA offers support, educational resources, and advocacy for those affected by eczema. They collaborate with healthcare professionals and researchers to promote awareness and improve outcomes for individuals with eczema.

American Academy of Dermatology (AAD):

While not exclusively focused on eczema, the AAD provides reliable information, guidelines, and resources related to dermatological conditions, including eczema. Their website is a valuable source for evidence-based information and advice.

Global Parents for Eczema Research (GPER):
GPER is an international organization dedicated to supporting parents of children with eczema. They aim to raise awareness, promote research, and provide a platform for parents to share experiences and advice.

Eczema Association of the Philippines:
This organization focuses on increasing awareness and providing support for individuals and families affected by eczema in the Philippines. They organize events, share educational materials, and foster a sense of community.

International Eczema Council (IEC):
The IEC brings together dermatologists, researchers, and healthcare professionals worldwide to collaborate on advancing eczema research, treatment, and education. Their work contributes to a global understanding of eczema and informs best practices in its management.

These support organizations contribute significantly to the eczema community by offering a range of services, from educational resources and advocacy to fostering connections among individuals facing similar challenges. Whether through online forums, local events, or research initiatives, these organizations play a vital role in improving the quality of life for those impacted by eczema.

Chapter 13

Skin care routine and diet

for curing eczema

Morning:

- Cleansing: Use a mild, fragrance-free cleanser to cleanse your face.

- Hydration: Apply a hypoallergenic, fragrance-free moisturizer to lock in hydration.
- Sun Protection: If going outside, use a broad-spectrum SPF 30 or higher sunscreen to protect your skin.

Diet

- Hydrate Inside and Out: Start your day with a glass of water. Follow your skincare routine, emphasizing gentle cleansing, moisturizing, and sun protection.
- Breakfast: Include foods rich in omega-3s like a serving of salmon or flaxseeds. Add antioxidant-rich fruits or vegetables to your meal.

Afternoon:

- Moisturize: Reapply moisturizer as needed, especially if your skin feels dry.

Diet

- Stay Hydrated: Continue drinking water throughout the day.
- Lunch: Opt for a well-balanced meal with lean protein (chicken, tofu), whole grains, and a variety of colorful vegetables.

Evening:

Diet only

- Dinner: Incorporate more omega-3s with another serving of fatty fish or plant-based sources. Include a mix of antioxidant-rich vegetables.
- Probiotics: If you enjoy fermented foods, consider having them as part of your dinner.

Night:
- Cleansing: Cleanse your face again with a gentle cleanser to remove impurities.
- Treatment (if prescribed): If your dermatologist has prescribed any specific treatments, apply them according to their instructions.
- Moisturize: Apply a richer moisturizer before bedtime to nourish your skin overnight.

Diet
- Hydrate: Drink a final glass of water.

CONCLUSION

In conclusion, understanding and managing eczema require a multifaceted approach that addresses the physical, emotional, and lifestyle aspects of this chronic skin condition. From the intricacies of its various types to the nuances of triggers, diagnostic processes, and diverse treatment modalities, individuals affected by eczema navigate a complex landscape. Throughout this journey, the significance of patient narratives, caregiver insights, and support organizations becomes evident, fostering a sense of community and empowerment.

As research continues to advance and innovative therapies emerge, the future of eczema management holds promise. The integration of personalized care, holistic approaches, and ongoing support systems is pivotal for enhancing the quality of life for those with eczema. Moreover, emphasizing mental health support, raising awareness, and promoting prevention strategies contribute to a comprehensive understanding of eczema beyond its visible symptoms.

The recommended readings, glossary, and resources provided offer individuals a toolkit to deepen their understanding, make informed decisions, and actively participate in their eczema management. As the eczema community continues to share experiences, advocate for research, and support one another, the collective journey becomes a testament to resilience and unity.

Continued advancements in research and ongoing collaborations among healthcare professionals, researchers, and support organizations promise to further illuminate the complexities of eczema. As scientific understanding deepens, so too will the array of targeted treatments and interventions, offering hope for more effective and personalized care.

The emotional and psychological impact of eczema cannot be overstated. Addressing these aspects, along with emphasizing the importance of mental health support and fostering a strong sense of community, contributes to a more compassionate and holistic approach to eczema care.

www.ingramcontent.com/pod-product-compliance
Lightning Source LLC
Chambersburg PA
CBHW070905250726

48662CB00003B/1518